Steven L.King

DEONTAY WILDER: THE UNYIELDING WARRIOR

Triumphs and trials of a heavyweight champion

Steven L.King

TABLE OF CONTENT

INTRODUCTION

One name reverberates through the annals of the sport in the brutal realm of heavyweight boxing, where resilience and strength collide: Deontay Wilder. "The Unyielding Warrior" explores the gripping story of a man whose adventure extends beyond the boxing ring. This book reveals the victories and setbacks that shaped Wilder's journey from impoverished origins to the height of heavyweight greatness. Wilder's story is proof of the unwavering spirit that drives him ahead and the tremendous strength of his fists—the indomitable determination that sets legends apart from competitors. Come along as we delve into the mind and spirit of a heavyweight champion—a man whose story goes beyond the mat and speaks to tenacity, selflessness, and unwavering resolve.

CHAPTER 1: WHO IS DEONTAY WILDER

American professional boxer Deontay Wilder was born on October 22, 1985, and he rose to prominence in the heavyweight category thanks to his potent hitting prowess and commanding presence. Originating from Tuscaloosa, Alabama, Wilder took up boxing at the age of 20, which was a rather late start to his career. His motivation for taking up boxing was to assist his daughter financially since she was born with spina bifida.

With a stellar amateur career that included an Olympic bronze in the heavyweight class in 2008, Wilder rapidly established himself. After going professional in 2008, he became well-known for his knockout abilities and his incredible knockout ratio, which captivated the boxing community. Referred to as "The Bronze Bomber," Wilder's potent right hand turned into his go-to tool, resulting in multiple knockouts and solidifying his reputation as a formidable opponent in the heavyweight division.

When Wilder defeated Bermane Stiverne in January 2015 to win the WBC heavyweight title, he officially became the champion of the WBC. He successfully defended his title several times, frequently displaying his powerful striking ability and unconventional boxing technique. Due to his perfect record and impressive knockouts, Wilder rose to the top of the heavyweight class.

When Wilder challenged British heavyweight Tyson Fury in December 2018, it was one of his most memorable battles. With a contentious split decision, Wilder was able to hold onto his WBC belt. In February 2020, Fury rescheduled the bout and emerged victorious, handing Wilder his first defeat as a professional. The bout created a gripping rivalry between the two competitors and attracted a lot of attention.

In addition to his prowess as a boxer, Wilder is known for his extravagant entrances into the ring, frequently donning ornate costumes, and his captivating demeanour. Additionally, he has been involved in a number of charitable endeavours, supporting them and utilising his position to spread the word about spina bifida.

Although Wilder's career in boxing has been filled with highs and lows, there is no denying his influence on the sport. The boxing world will never forget his status as a knockout artist and one of the most formidable heavyweights of his time.

CHAPTER 2: EARLY YEARS AND ENTRY INTO BOXING

Deontay Wilder grew up in a working-class family in Tuscaloosa, Alabama, and experienced a variety of hardships. When his daughter Naieya was born in 2005 with spina bifida, his life took a dramatic shift, motivating him to take up boxing as a way to support his family financially.

At the age of 20, Wilder began boxing relatively late, but his innate agility and talent were evident right away. He started a voyage that would determine his future in the sport at Skyy Boxing Gym in Northport, Alabama, under the tutelage of coach Jay Deas.

Wilder's commitment to hard work and quick advancement at the amateur level paid off when he won a bronze medal in the heavyweight class at the 2008 Beijing Olympics. His ascent to the top of the boxing world helped him establish himself and provide a better future for his family.

2008 saw Wilder turn professional, and his early bouts

demonstrated both his raw power and knockout prowess. His aggressive approach and impressive knockout percentage earned him the opportunity to challenge for the WBC heavyweight title. After defeating Bermane Stiverne in January 2015, Wilder became the first American to win a world heavyweight title in almost ten years.

Motivated by self-interest and a desire to support his family, Wilder entered the boxing world, setting the stage for his eventual influence in the heavyweight class.

Throughout his boxing career, Wilder exhibited tenacity and resolve. Boxing provided structure and discipline, which helped him find purpose and comfort in a harsh environment where he grew up. His experiences as a young father gave him the motivation to turn his physical prowess into a professional career.

Coach Jay Deas helped Wilder develop his unconventional approach and devastating punches, which became his signature. His quick ascent through the amateur ranks, which resulted in a bronze medal at the Olympics, suggested the promise that would eventually shape his professional career.

In his professional career, boxing circles were abuzz with talk of Wilder's knockout ability. His wins were not only magnificent demonstrations of his ability to finish fights with a single, devastating blow. Together with his unusual demeanour and spectacular ring entrances, the charming and gregarious Wilder also attracted notice for his showmanship, which enhanced his skill in the ring. Outside of athletics, Wilder has been involved in philanthropy, donating to numerous humanitarian projects and using his platform to spread knowledge of spina bifida. His dedication to giving back reveals a side of him that remains hidden in the boxing ring.

In addition to illustrating a personal tale of overcoming hardship, Wilder's early years and foray into boxing also demonstrate the life-changing potential of sports. The determination and enthusiasm that characterised his formative years in the boxing world are evident in his influence on the heavyweight class and the sport overall.

CHAPTER 3: RISE THROUGH THE RANKS

The ascent of professional boxer Deontay Wilder was nothing short of spectacular. His early bouts after going professional in 2008 demonstrated his extraordinary strength and distinct fighting style. With a string of knockout wins, Wilder's perfect record attracted notice from the boxing community right away.

When Wilder fought Bermane Stiverne for the WBC heavyweight title in January 2015, it was one of the major turning points in his career. In addition to earning the coveted title, the victory made him the first American to win a heavyweight world championship in almost ten years.

Throughout his title tenure, Wilder successfully defended the title against a number of opponents, each of whom brought attention to his lethal right hand and capacity for early finish times. In addition to his knockout skills, his charm and self-assurance outside the ring helped him become more well-known in the boxing community.

In December 2018, one of the biggest events in Wilder's career was the much-awaited fight with Tyson Fury. Although the fight finished in a contentious split draw, it thrust Wilder into the public eye. Even though it was Wilder's first professional defeat, the rematch in February 2020 cemented his place in the heavyweight category as a household star.

As he rose through the ranks, Wilder demonstrated both his knockout strength and his capacity to captivate the crowd. His captivating demeanour, combined with his unbeaten record, gave him a powerful presence in the heavyweight division. Even if losses and disappointments are inevitable in any career, Wilder's ascent through the ranks is nevertheless evidence of his influence on the game and his capacity to enthral spectators worldwide.

CHAPTER 4: DEONTAY WILDER FIGHTING STYLE

The former heavyweight champion of the WBC, Deontay Wilder, is renowned for his distinct and powerful fighting style. His remarkable strength, especially in his right hand, is one of his most defining characteristics and has earned him the moniker "The Bronze Bomber." With a strong knockout ratio, Wilder has demonstrated his ability to terminate bouts quickly with devastating punches.

Unlike many other professional boxers, Wilder began boxing rather late in life, which contributes to his unconventional background. His innate athleticism and sheer punching power helped him rise through the ranks fast, even with his scant amateur experience.

At 6 feet 7 inches tall and with an 83-inch reach, one of Wilder's greatest assets is his extraordinary reach. He sets up his strong right hand and successfully uses his long arms to keep opponents at a distance. He uses his jab both offensively to set up his power shots and defensively to maintain distance, making it a crucial part of his game.

Despite critiques of his footwork lacking polish compared to some of his peers, Wilder's aggressive style is enhanced by it. He moves horizontally most of the time, using sudden bursts of speed to get closer as needed. He can seize opportunities fast with this technique, especially when opponents don't anticipate his mobility.

Wilder's signature weapon is his right hand, which he throws with stunning force. His blows have a startling pace that often catches opponents off guard. His technique is a fast, looping action. Numerous opponents have found it difficult to withstand the strength of Wilder's right hand, as demonstrated by his knockout victories.

But as seen by his debut fight against Tyson Fury, Wilder's reliance on his right hand has occasionally left him exposed. Despite having a formidable arsenal, some contend that he is not as versatile as other elite heavyweights. His defensive techniques and boxing prowess have come under scrutiny, especially when up against opponents with formidable skill sets overall. Rather than using more conventional defensive strategies, Wilder prefers to use his quickness and elusive moves. Though, as some of his most difficult fights have shown, this strategy has often served him well, it also leaves him open to counterattacks.

Deontay Wilder's striking prowess, unconventional upbringing, and dependence on a dominant right hand characterise his fighting style. Despite lacking some of the elegance of previous heavyweight champions, he is still a strong force in the division thanks to his ability to terminate matches decisively. Sophisticating his techniques and adjusting to new opponents will be essential for him to succeed at the top of the professional boxing ranks as he advances in his career.

The main goal of Wilder's offensive approach is to create gaps for his lethal right hand. He frequently employs his jab to conceal the timing of his potent straight right in addition to using it as a rangefinder. Many heavyweights find him to be a difficult opponent because of his unpredictable nature and capacity for surprise attacks. Resilience is another noteworthy feature of Wilder's fighting technique. He has proven in multiple fights that he is capable of taking hits and still fighting by using his resolve and willpower. In his debut battle against Tyson Fury, he showed off his tenacity by surviving a knockdown and finishing the fight.

Not only can Wilder knock people out with his right hand, but his left hook and uppercut are also very effective strikers. Even though he might not use these punches as much, they are nonetheless quite effective and give his offensive arsenal a surprising element that makes it more difficult for opponents to predict his strikes.

However, there have been controversial and unsuccessful times in Wilder's boxing career. Tyson Fury exposed Wilder's technical shortcomings in the rematch, particularly in terms of head movement and defence techniques. Critics contend that against players with well-rounded skill sets, Wilder may have difficulties due to his weak defensive base.

Wilder's mental toughness and unwavering attitude have played a significant role in his success. His belief in his ability to change the course of a fight with a single blow and his unwavering attitude have helped him to many comeback triumphs.

Wilder is renowned for having extraordinary athleticism and conditioning. Due to his endurance, he has been able to stay in multiple battles to the end and keep up his strength into later rounds, which makes him a more formidable opponent.

It will be crucial for Wilder to modify and improve his methods as he advances in his career, particularly when facing opponents who take advantage of his flaws. How well he performs against elite heavyweight opponents will decide his legacy in the sport of boxing. Fans and commentators alike continue to find Wilder's journey to be fascinating as he looks to reclaim the heavyweight title and establish his legacy in the sport.

CHAPTER 5: PROFESSIONAL DEBUT

On November 15, 2008, in Nashville, Tennessee, American boxer Deontay Wilder made his professional debut against Ethan Cox. The fight was the first of Wilder's adventures in the heavyweight boxing scene, where he would go on to become well-known.

With an excellent amateur record that included a bronze medal at the Beijing Olympics in 2008, Wilder made a successful transition into the professional boxing world. His entry into the professional ranks sparked a lot of interest because he had a reputation as a strong and captivating fighter.

In his debut, Wilder quickly displayed his devastating punching power against Ethan Cox. In the first round, he won by technical knockout in just 44 seconds. This swift and convincing victory demonstrated Wilder's exceptional knockout power and set the tone for his early professional career.

Wilder's knockout streak garnered attention and parallels to boxing greats as he continued to improve his professional record. Many attributed Wilder's success in the ring to his distinctive style, characterised by a powerful right hand and unorthodox yet effective approaches.

Over the next few years, Wilder rose through the heavyweight ranks and developed a solid reputation as a knockout fighter. His ability to end contests with a single blow enthralled fans, making him a formidable opponent in the boxing world.

It's crucial to remember that Wilder's professional debut signalled the start of the path that would eventually take him to the WBC heavyweight championship. He became a prominent figure in the sport thanks to his knockout victories, charm, and undefeated record, which paved the way for high-profile bouts and made him one of the best heavyweights of his time.

Despite setbacks in his career, including his first professional defeat to Tyson Fury in 2020, Wilder's debut is still a pivotal point in his narrative. It represents the arrival of a strong athlete in the world of professional boxing, portending a significant career that will play out in the years to come.

After his triumphant debut, Deontay Wilder's early professional career showcased a run of commanding victories that highlighted his incredible punching power. Boxing fans and commentators took notice of his quick rise up the ranks as he kept compiling an outstanding record.

As opponents were unable to withstand the force of Wilder's right hand, his knockout streak became a defining characteristic of his fights. He was a fascinating presence in the heavyweight class thanks to his exceptional mix of strength, speed, and athleticism.

As Wilder faced a range of opponents with different approaches, it was clear how adaptive and resilient he was. His win over Kelvin Price in December 2012 was a significant turning point in his early career. In spite of hardships and an early knockdown in the bout, Wilder demonstrated his tenacity by returning to win by knockout in the third round.

For Wilder, the fight against Bermane Stiverne for the WBC heavyweight championship in 2015 proved to be crucial. In what was a major turning point in his career, Wilder put on a strong performance to win the fight by unanimous decision and capture the championship. With his reign as heavyweight champion, Wilder cemented his place in the heavyweight class. His later defences, which included noteworthy wins against opponents like Chris Arreola and Artur Szpilka, solidified his reputation as a formidable opponent. Although Wilder's run of knockout victories eventually ended in 2020 with a draw and subsequent defeat to Tyson Fury, his professional debut remains a significant moment in his career. It was the springboard for a career that showcased his rise from Olympic bronze medalist to world champion, bringing thrills and surprises to the heavyweight stage. Wilder's impact on the sport is still felt today, leaving behind an enduring legacy in the annals of boxing history.

CHAPTER 6: NOTABLE VICTORIES

Deontay Wilder, known as "The Bronze Bomber," has had an incredible boxing career highlighted by his noteworthy wins. On January 17, 2015, he defeated Bermane Stiverne to win the WBC heavyweight title, which was one of his most notable victories. Being the first American to win a world heavyweight title in almost ten years, Wilder won via unanimous decision after showcasing his strength and accuracy throughout the bout.

In March 2018, Wilder achieved yet another noteworthy victory in his career by successfully defending his WBC title against Luis Ortiz. Wilder demonstrated his knockout power and resilience in the face of hardship and being pushed to the limit by stopping Ortiz in the tenth round. This triumph proved that he was a formidable heavyweight fighter and cemented his reputation as such.

In May 2019, one of the most remarkable triumphs in Wilder's career occurred when he decisively defeated

Dominic Breazeale. In the opening round, Wilder's powerful right hand put a stop to the battle, which lasted less than two minutes. With this victory, Wilder further cemented his reputation as a deadly force in the heavyweight class and displayed his powerful punching ability.

In November 2019, in a much-awaited rematch with Luis Ortiz, Wilder encountered hardship once more. Even though Ortiz outclassed him for the majority of the fight, Wilder emerged victorious in a thrilling round by demonstrating his tenacity and knockout power. This victory demonstrated Wilder's capacity to change the course of a fight with a single, potent blow.

The battle that took place in December 2018 between Deontay Wilder and Tyson Fury was one of the most talked-about bouts in recent memory. Despite the disputed draw that resulted from the battle, Wilder's knockdowns of Fury demonstrated his ability to influence the outcome of the fight. However, the passionate nature of their rematch in February 2020 cemented Wilder's standing as a top heavyweight, despite the bouts ending in a draw.

All of these wins demonstrate Deontay Wilder's tenacity, knockout power, and capacity to prevail in trying circumstances. Even though he has had several hiccups in his career, his memorable wins have surely made a lasting impression on the heavyweight boxing community.

Deontay Wilder and Tyson Fury squared up in a much-awaited rematch for the WBC heavyweight belt in February 2020. Even though Fury was able to stop the fight in the seventh round, it demonstrated Wilder's determination to take on difficult challenges. The fight demonstrated Wilder's spirit and tenacity in the face of loss.

A pivotal point in Wilder's career was his victory over Luis Ortiz in their first meeting in March 2018. Despite Ortiz being regarded as one of the most proficient and lethal opponents in the division, Wilder showcased his resilience and striking power by winning via knockout. One notable victory earlier in Wilder's career was over Chris Arreola in July 2016. In spite of suffering a broken right hand and a torn bicep during the bout, Wilder showed incredible bravery and tenacity to win by stoppage in the eighth round. This triumph demonstrated his capacity to overcome obstacles in the ring, including physical challenges.

In January 2015, Wilder achieved another noteworthy victory by effectively defending his WBC belt against opponent Eric Molina. In the ninth round, Wilder won via knockout after dominating the contest. This victory demonstrated his steady ability to end fights and keep his perfect record.

Deontay Wilder's career has been filled with both successes and setbacks, but his memorable wins have cemented his reputation as one of the most formidable and captivating heavyweights of all time. Whether it's through impressive knockouts or tough decisions, Wilder's exploits in the ring have endeared him to boxing fans and solidified his position as one of the heavyweight division's finest.

CHAPTER 7: MENTAL TOUGHNESS

Deontay Wilder, the former WBC heavyweight champion, widely impresses with his exceptional mental toughness inside the boxing ring. One key aspect of his mental resilience is his unwavering self-belief. Wilder exudes confidence, often expressing an unshakable belief in his abilities and predicting victory with conviction. This confidence has been a driving force throughout his career, allowing him to overcome challenges and setbacks.

Another element contributing to Wilder's mental toughness is his ability to maintain focus and composure under pressure. In the heat of intense boxing matches, he remains calm and strategic, showcasing a disciplined mindset. This mental composure is crucial in high-stakes situations, enabling him to stay focused on his game plan even when facing formidable opponents.

Wilder's resilience in the face of adversity is evident in his comeback victories. One notable example is his first fight against Luis Ortiz, where he faced adversity in the seventh round but rallied back to secure a knockout win. This ability to bounce back from difficult situations showcases his mental fortitude and determination. Wilder's approach to training and preparation reflects his mental toughness. He is known for his rigorous training regimen and dedication to honing his skills. This disciplined work ethic demonstrates a commitment to mental and physical conditioning, essential for success at the highest levels of professional boxing.

It's essential to acknowledge that mental toughness in boxing also involves dealing with criticism and handling the pressure of expectations. Wilder has faced criticism, particularly after his loss to Tyson Fury, but he has maintained a positive mindset and expressed a strong desire to learn and improve from his experiences. Deontay Wilder's mental toughness is a multi-faceted trait encompassing self-belief, composure under pressure, resilience, and a disciplined approach to training. These characteristics have played a significant role in his success and have solidified his standing as one of the top heavyweight boxers in the world.

Furthermore, Wilder's mental toughness shines through

as he continuously adapts and evolves. Throughout his career, he has showcased a willingness to learn from each fight, adjusting his strategies and refining his techniques. This adaptability speaks to his mental flexibility, a crucial aspect of resilience in the dynamic and unpredictable world of professional boxing.

Facing defeat against Tyson Fury, Wilder exhibited grace under pressure by accepting the loss and expressing a determination to bounce back stronger. Instead of dwelling on setbacks, he channelled his energy into self-improvement and prepared for the rematch. This ability to turn adversity into motivation highlights his mental strength and forward-thinking mindset.

Wilder's mental toughness is evident in his ability to handle the spotlight and the immense expectations that come with being a high-profile athlete. The pressure of being a heavyweight champion is immense, yet Wilder has consistently faced it head-on, demonstrating mental resilience in the face of both external pressures and internal challenges.

Beyond the physical demands of the sport, mental toughness is crucial in dealing with the psychological aspects of boxing. Wilder's intimidating presence in the ring and his unyielding self-confidence play a significant role in affecting the psyche of his opponents. This mental edge can influence the dynamics of a fight, as opponents may find themselves mentally fatigued or hesitant when confronted with Wilder's unwavering resolve.

Deontay Wilder's mental toughness extends beyond his physical abilities, encompassing a holistic approach to the mental aspects of boxing. His capacity to adapt, learn from setbacks, handle pressure, and maintain a strong mindset positions him as not only a formidable competitor in the heavyweight division but also as a testament to the importance of mental fortitude in the world of professional sports.

CHAPTER 8: TRIAL AND CHALLENGES

Throughout his professional boxing career, former WBC heavyweight champion Deontay Wilder has experienced both victories and setbacks. In December 2018, Wilder faced one of the most significant challenges of his life: his first meeting with Tyson Fury. Despite Wilder's remarkable record of knockouts, Fury held on to avoid two knockdowns and secure a contentious split decision. This posed a serious problem for Wilder since it cast doubt on his capacity to outclass elite opponents.

The rematch between Wilder and Fury in February 2020 was another crucial turning point in Wilder's career. This time, the outcome was different for Wilder, as he lost via TKO in the seventh round. The loss exposed flaws in both Wilder's boxing approach and strategy, as Fury's aggressive style took advantage of gaps in Wilder's defence. In addition to ending Wilder's lengthy tenure as the WBC champion, the defeat forced him to reevaluate and drastically change his strategy.

The "Bronze Bomber," Wilder, has faced challenges as

well as benefits from his dependence on his strong right hand. Even though it resulted in multiple knockouts and wins, it also revealed a weakness that opponents could exploit if they managed to neutralise that weapon. The rematch between Wilder and Tyson Fury highlighted the necessity for him to have a more varied skill set, including better defensive and footwork skills.

Outside of the ring, Wilder has encountered difficulties in negotiations and contract conflicts. Legal issues obstructed his plans for a trilogy matchup with Fury, making his return to championship contention much more difficult. In addition to putting Wilder's willpower to the test, these contractual difficulties had an impact on his public perception and relationships with several boxing industry players.

Deontay Wilder is still a powerful force in the heavyweight class despite his failures, and his career is proof of how unpredictable the world of professional boxing can be. He has had to change as a boxer as a result of his experiences, both psychologically and physically. It remains to be seen if Wilder can overcome these obstacles and win another world championship, but his tenacity and willpower imply that he is far from done leaving his mark on the sport.

Apart from the difficulties in the ring, Deontay Wilder has also been the target of criticism and controversy for remarks and actions he has taken outside of boxing contests. His fiery temper and audacious remarks, especially in the moments before fights, have occasionally attracted criticism as well as attention. This facet of Wilder's character has influenced how fans and the media view him, giving his public persona an additional degree of complexity.

Following the second Fury bout, Wilder openly voiced his displeasure with his old trainer, Mark Breland, which led to more difficulties. The choice to end the fight early caused tension between Wilder and Breland, which resulted in a public altercation. This division sparked concerns about Wilder's team's stability and potential effects on his performance moving forward.

Controversy arose from Wilder's reaction to his defeat against Fury, which included claims of dirty work and wearing a bulky outfit that affected his legs prior to the bout. Although these kinds of statements can be a part of boxing's mental warfare, they also sparked scepticism and discussions concerning sportsmanship and responsibility in defeat.

Both supporters and detractors of Wilder closely monitor his progress as he overcomes these obstacles, curious to see how he adjusts and bounces back from failures. The heavyweight class is notoriously unpredictable, and Wilder's struggles serve as a stark reminder of how cruel professional boxing can be—a single blow or a calculated move can mean the difference between success and failure.

Deontay Wilder's tenacity and resolve remain important focuses despite these difficulties. In the end, how he handles setbacks, adjusts as needed, and stays competitive will determine how his career develops in the later stages. Whether it's about getting a rematch with Fury or going after other prospects in the heavyweight division, Wilder's story continues to be one of great interest in the exciting world of professional boxing.

8.1 SET BACK AND DEFEATS

Throughout his boxing career, Deontay Wilder has faced obstacles and losses that have moulded his path in the sport. A significant obstacle he faced was his defeat by Tyson Fury in February 2020. In the fight, Wilder lost for the first time as a professional, which was a major turning point in his career.

Following a contentious stalemate in their first encounter, the boxers faced defeat against Fury. Often referred to as the "Bronze Bomber," Wilder's strong right hand has been the decisive factor in several of his prior battles, resulting in knockout victories. Nonetheless, Fury's tactical approach and capacity to withstand Wilder's blows revealed several flaws in the American boxer's repertoire.

The rematch between Wilder and Fury in October 2021 was another blow. Even though Wilder was determined to get the championship back, he lost again, this time by knockout in the eleventh round. The defeat prompted concerns about Wilder's flexibility and his capacity to modify his strategy while facing opponents with disparate playing styles.

Wilder's dependence on his strong right hand had proven to be a double-edged sword throughout his career. Although it helped him win a lot of fights, opponents like Fury took advantage of this predictability to cause him to lose and suffer setbacks. The losses also sparked discussions about improving his boxing technique and building a more diverse skill set.

Some have attributed Wilder's setbacks to injuries. During the Fury rematch, it was discovered that Wilder had sustained a bicep injury. Injuries can greatly impact a boxer's performance, hindering their capacity to carry out their strategy.

It is impossible to ignore Wilder's tenacity and will in the face of these obstacles. In sports, losses are common, and many legendary boxers have suffered setbacks before rising back stronger. Fans and commentators will be keenly following Wilder's post-defeat path to see how he grows, changes, and absorbs these experiences to prepare for a triumphant return to the competitive heavyweight boxing scene.

Wilder's losses have also spurred debate about his

coaching staff and corner. There were discussions on Fury's coaching staff's contribution to getting him ready for his opponents' difficulties following the second fight. Others questioned if Wilder needed to bring in new ideas and tactics from those in his corner.

In addition, it's important to recognize the psychological effects of losing a game after another. Known for his bold and self-assured style, Wilder encountered a new mental obstacle following setbacks. In order to win back the title and establish oneself in the division, a boxer must overcome the psychological effects of losses. Following the Fury defeats, Wilder made good on his contractual demand for a third fight, indicating his intention to make up for the earlier outcomes. The much-awaited trilogy fight demonstrated Wilder's will to turn his career around. But whether that battle ended in victory or defeat, the story of his career would surely be further shaped by the result.

It is important to remember that failures and setbacks are a natural part of the path for any athlete, and they frequently act as stimulants for development. The way that Wilder handles hardship will determine his legacy in the game. In the cutthroat world of heavyweight boxing, his ability to grow from his mistakes, modify his approach, and plug the holes left by his opponents will be crucial to his success going forward.

8.2 INJURY STRUGGLES

Throughout his career, Deontay Wilder has struggled with injuries, especially after losing to Tyson Fury in February 2020, his first professional fight. The most prominent wound was a bicep injury that Wilder disclosed before the bout, citing his training camp as the source of the injury.

It was unclear if Wilder's bicep ailment affected how well he performed in the ring against Fury. While some critics contend that the injury might have played a role in his disappointing performance, others think it might have led to his struggles adjusting to Fury's unconventional approach.

Apart from the injury to his bicep, Wilder has experienced issues with his ear in the rematch with Fury. There have been rumours that Wilder's eardrum burst during the bout, which may have affected his balance and equilibrium. Such ailments can significantly impact a boxer's ability to perform at their peak, especially when facing a skilled opponent like Tyson Fury.

For Wilder, recovering from these injuries has probably been difficult. It has required a lot of training and therapy to restore strength and make sure he is in top shape for fights in the future. A professional athlete's journey always includes overcoming physical hurdles, and Wilder's tenacity in the face of these difficulties demonstrates his will to regain his position in the heavyweight class.

CHAPTER 9: TRIUMPHS ON THE WORLD STAGE

Over his stellar career, Deontay Wilder has achieved multiple victories on the international scene. Among his noteworthy accomplishments is his incredible knockout record, which has earned him the moniker "The Bronze Bomber." Contributing to his success, Wilder's strong right hand has been a dominant force in the boxing world.

A notable victory for Wilder occurred in January 2015 when he fought for the WBC heavyweight title against Bermane Stiverne. Wilder won via unanimous decision after repeatedly taking Stiverne to the canvas thanks to his remarkable punching power. Being the first American to win a world heavyweight title in almost ten years, Wilder's victory was a pivotal point in his career. With two triumphant title defences, Wilder maintained his stellar record and demonstrated his ability to end fights with decisiveness. One notable fight is his 2018 matchup with Luis Ortiz, in which Wilder overcame hardships to produce an incredible knockout in the tenth round. This triumph demonstrated not only his strength but also his fortitude and capacity to deal with difficult opponents.

Wilder and Tyson Fury squared off in a much-awaited rematch in 2020. Despite the fact that the fight was a draw, it prepared them for their rematch in February 2020. Even though he lost the fight in the end, Wilder showed incredible bravery and tenacity by getting back up after Fury knocked him down. In addition to showcasing Wilder's unwavering spirit, this fight cemented his reputation as a heavyweight fighter. Despite the difficulties posed by the Fury trilogy, Wilder has had a tremendous overall influence on global affairs. Fans all across the world respect and admire him for the unforgettable impression that his thrilling performances and knockout wins have made on the sport. Notwithstanding obstacles, Wilder's career in the heavyweight class has been a monument to his strength, power, and fortitude, securing his place in boxing history.

Outside of the boxing ring, Deontay Wilder's victories on

the global scene have a positive cultural and economic influence on the sport. He is well-known in the sports and entertainment industries thanks to his captivating fighting style and captivating personality.

Wilder's ascent to prominence rekindled interest in the heavyweight class. Being one of the most gregarious and vocal fighters in the sport, he invigorated the heavyweight scene and attracted a worldwide following. His captivating demeanour and knockout ability helped boxing regain the interest of the general public.

It is impossible to overstate Wilder's influence on boxing's business environment. His highly publicised fights generated large pay-per-view sales and attendance figures, which boosted the sport's bottom line. His fights became big sporting events, bringing in a lot of money and improving boxing's standing overall, especially when he faced well-known opponents like Tyson Fury. Wilder's accomplishments also enabled the greater international recognition of American heavyweights. During a time when foreign boxers frequently ruled the heavyweight division, Wilder's accomplishments restored interest in American boxing and instilled a

feeling of patriotism among supporters.
Notwithstanding the difficulties and disappointments he
encountered, Wilder's influence goes beyond the
scoreboard. His journey has been one of tenacity,
resolve, and fortitude, captivating the interest of
supporters and motivating a new wave of boxers. Even
though Wilder hasn't won any of his recent fights, his
legacy in the sports world is still very much intact, and
he has left a lasting impression on the history of
heavyweight boxing.

CHAPTER 10: OUTSIDE THE RING

Outside of the boxing arena, Deontay Wilder has achieved great success and shown a diverse personality in addition to his potent blows. A noteworthy feature of Wilder's non-playing life is his dedication to charitable giving. He has actively supported topics pertaining to children, education, and healthcare through a variety of charitable projects.

Wilder demonstrates his commitment to assisting others by actively participating in charitable activities and community outreach initiatives. He has emphasised the value of giving back and having a good influence outside of the boxing ring by using his platform to generate money and awareness for charities that support poor communities.

Apart from his charitable endeavours, Deontay Wilder has looked into career prospects in the entertainment sector. In order to promote his life story and viewpoints, he has partnered with multiple media sources, made cameos on television shows, and taken part in documentaries. Beyond the intensity of the boxing ring, this venture into entertainment not only expands his fan base but also gives him a more intimate connection. Beyond boxing, Wilder's sense of style has grown to be a significant part of his public persona. His unique and frequently extravagant style has highlighted him in fashion journals and established him as a fashion icon. With his involvement in the fashion industry, Wilder's public persona has taken on a new dimension that highlights his uniqueness and inventiveness.

Speaking out on social issues such as racial inequity and justice, Deontay Wilder has used his platform. He has contributed to the larger discussions about social justice by passionately voicing his thoughts on these issues outside of the boxing world.

Outside of the ring, Deontay Wilder demonstrates a complex person who is not just defined by his boxing successes. Through his humanitarian pursuits, entertainment enterprises, and vocal social activism, Wilder has effectively developed a multifaceted public persona that appeals to a global fan base.

Deontay Wilder is a businessman who has dabbled in

entrepreneurship, building his own company and brand. In addition to his boxing career, Wilder has shown a strong desire to leave a lasting legacy through business collaborations, product endorsements, and the creation of his own line of items. His financial future is not only secured by this business mentality, but it also enables him to take advantage of his marketability and popularity.

Through his activities outside of the ring, Wilder has demonstrated his dedication to health and fitness. He has been a strong proponent of leading a healthy lifestyle and frequently provides his social media followers with exercise plans, dietary advice, and inspirational sayings. Wilder's emphasis on well-being positions him as a positive influence in this arena, aligning with the growing trend of athletes supporting physical and mental wellness.

In the field of education, Deontay Wilder has participated in programs that encourage and mentor youth. He has utilised his experiences to inspire people to follow their aspirations and emphasises the significance of education, hard work, perseverance, and dedication.

When it comes to his media presence, Wilder has made use of social media to engage with his audience directly and provide details about his personal life, workout regimens, and behind-the-scenes activities. He has been able to break down the barriers between the audience and the athlete by developing more personal contact with them thanks to this direct engagement.

It's important to note that Wilder has faced difficulties on his path outside of the ring. His ability to bounce back from setbacks—both inside and outside of the boxing ring—further contributes to the story of a fighter who welcomes hardship and turns it into an opportunity for self-improvement.

Aside from boxing, Deontay Wilder is involved in a variety of endeavours, including philanthropy, entertainment, fashion, business, fitness, education, and social advocacy. This all-encompassing outlook on life outside of boxing presents a well-rounded person who is defined by his efforts to make a positive impact on many aspects of society rather than just his sporting accomplishments.

10.1 PERSONAL LIFE

Deontay Wilder became well-known for his strong punches and outstanding knockout percentage. Raised in Tuscaloosa, Alabama, Wilder first went for a career in basketball and football before realising at the age of twenty that he had boxing potential.

Among the difficulties of Wilder's early life was learning that his daughter had spina bifida. His desire for boxing success sprang from his personal adversity, which motivated him to give his family a better existence. Compared to many other boxers, he entered the sport somewhat later, but his innate athleticism and commitment helped him rise through the ranks quickly. When Deontay Wilder placed third in the heavyweight division at the 2008 Beijing Olympics, it was the beginning of his big break. This accomplishment acted as a springboard for his formally launched professional career later that year. Renowned as "The Bronze Bomber," Wilder was able to finish opponents in the first round of fights thanks to his tremendous knockout power.

After fighting Bermane Stiverne in 2015, Wilder won the WBC heavyweight title, which he successfully defended on several occasions. His flawless record, combined with his impressive knockout streak, made him a dangerous competitor in the heavyweight class.

Although Wilder's career took off, his private life came under investigation due to scandals involving his candid remarks and conflicts with other boxers, most notably Tyson Fury. In February 2020, after a fierce rivalry that lasted for a long time, Wilder lost his first fight as a professional. The fight was controversial; afterward, Wilder claimed that Fury had used foul play and cited problems with his training camp.

Despite obstacles, Deontay Wilder continues to have a profound impact on boxing history. His remarkable rise from a late starter to an Olympic medalist and world champion has left an enduring impression on the sport. It might be wise to investigate more recent sources for any developments on Deontay Wilder's life and career as of my last knowledge update in January 2022.

Deontay Wilder's charitable endeavours have defined his private existence. Motivated by his daughter's struggle with spina bifida, he has been actively involved in humanitarian work, particularly raising awareness and finances for children with disabilities. Because of his dedication to changing the world through beneficial causes outside of boxing, Wilder has gained the respect of his audience and shown a caring side of himself. Popularity was aided by Wilder's distinct style and persona, which were evident both inside and outside the ring. During public engagements, he frequently embraced his Southern heritage and had a captivating and colourful personality. This brought entertainment value to his boxing career and drew a wide range of supporters.

Even though Wilder's career was marred by disappointments, like the defeat to Tyson Fury described before, he persevered and declared his intention to win back the title. The controversy surrounding his loss stoked talk about possible rematches and his future tactics, which kept fans excited for when he would go back into the ring.

Wilder has dabbled in a number of business endeavours outside of boxing, such as acting and endorsements. His charismatic demeanour has made connections and exposed his adaptability and aspirations outside of the squared circle, opening doors to options beyond the sport.

10.2 PHILANTHROPY AND CONTRIBUTIONS

In addition to his skills in the boxing ring, Deontay Wilder has demonstrated a strong dedication to philanthropy and giving back to his community. One noteworthy aspect of Wilder's charity activities is his participation in projects that help underprivileged children and families. The boxer has expressed a strong desire to use his position to change things outside of the ring.

Wilder has ties to a number of philanthropic groups and programs that promote health, wellness, and education. His contributions frequently go toward initiatives that support young empowerment, offer educational opportunities, and help people who are struggling financially. Wilder's dedication to charity is a reflection of his conviction that he should use his fortune to help others—especially the most disadvantaged.

Supporting activities pertaining to health and wellness is one important area in which Wilder has had a long-lasting influence. Being well-known, he is conscious of the value of encouraging healthy living and has participated in events and campaigns to increase public awareness of a range of health-related concerns. Beyond the ring, Wilder's contributions positively impact several people, whether via fundraising endeavours or active involvement.

Furthermore, Wilder has a history of interacting personally with members of his community. His interactions with fans, particularly the younger ones, frequently convey strength and inspiration. Through his personal path and experiences, Wilder hopes to inspire people to overcome obstacles and follow their passions. It is noteworthy that although Deontay Wilder's charitable endeavours are not as well-known as his boxing career, his dedication to giving back is clear in a number of ways. Like many sportsmen who understand the positive influence they may have off the field (or, in this case, off the ring), Wilder has demonstrated through his contributions a desire to improve society and a sense of social duty.

Beyond the ring, Deontay Wilder's charitable initiatives and involvement in the community highlight a deeper dedication to improving the lives of others. Through his involvement in the community and his support of humanitarian causes, Wilder is a prime example of how athletes can play a significant role as social change agents.

Deontay Wilder has shown a special interest in family- and child-related humanitarian endeavours. His emphasis on youth-beneficial efforts frequently entails funding educational initiatives and projects meant to open doors for disadvantaged kids. Through his work in this area, Wilder has demonstrated his commitment to creating a better future for coming generations.

It is well known that Wilder plans and takes part in community-beneficial events. Through the coordination of charity matches, fundraisers, or collaboration with well-established groups, he proactively looks for methods to direct money to the most deserving. This practical approach to generosity shows a sincere desire to actually improve the lives of those who are struggling. Wilder has made contributions to humanitarian operations following disasters. He has always been the first to offer assistance during catastrophes, whether they be local issues or natural disasters, and he has used his platform to inspire others to pitch in as well. This shows a global view of generosity and a sense of responsibility that extends beyond his local community.

Deontay Wilder has a broad charitable background that includes work in the fields of health, education, community development, and disaster relief. In addition to being a strong boxer, his dedication to making significant contributions to society presents him as a socially conscious guy working to bring about positive change on a larger scale.

CHAPTER 11: LEGACY AND IMPACT

One well-known person in the realm of professional boxing is Deontay Wilder. Recognized for his remarkable strength and capacity for knockouts, Wilder has had a significant impact on the sport.

Wilder's influence on boxing is evident in his Olympic performance. At the 2008 Beijing Olympics, he proved his mettle on the global scene by winning a bronze medal in the heavyweight class. This early success served as a springboard for his 2008 start in the professional world.

Wilder's outstanding knockout record is among his greatest achievements in the game. Known by the nickname "The Bronze Bomber," he gained notoriety for his devastating right hand, which contributed to an astounding amount of knockouts. Fans were ecstatic, and this helped to make Wilder one of the most feared heavyweights of the recent past.

2015 saw Wilder overcome Bermane Stiverne to win the WBC heavyweight championship. He held the title for a number of years and won several well-known fights to successfully defend it. His legendary bouts with Tyson Fury and Luis Ortiz cemented his legacy in boxing history even further.

Wilder's influence goes beyond the ring since he came to represent tenacity and willpower. He overcame personal obstacles and disappointments, such as a delayed start to boxing and health problems, to show how persistence is key to success.

But Wilder's first-ever professional defeat to Tyson Fury in February 2020 also leaves a lasting impression on history. Even though it was a setback, the loss demonstrated his sportsmanship and humility in accepting defeat. This period of his career underlines the unpredictability of the game and the value of grace in both win and defeat, which adds another level of complexity to his legacy.

The influence of Wilder extends beyond his accomplishments in the ring. His captivating fighting style and captivating personality helped heavyweight boxing become more popular overall. His entry into the division restored excitement and attention to a weight class that had suffered from a lack of star power in the past.

In the future, Deontay Wilder will be regarded as a formidable and exciting fighter who left a lasting impression on the heavyweight class. His contributions to the sport, both in terms of his fighting technique and personal journey, will continue to influence and motivate future boxers for many generations to come.

The influence that Wilder has had on boxing goes beyond numbers and trophies. In addition to the sport, he has influenced the larger cultural and social milieu. As an African American athlete, Wilder rose to prominence and served as an example to many aspiring combatants, especially those who were up against hardship. His accomplishments and tenacity dispelled stereotypes, demonstrating that one's background should not restrict one's ability in the world of professional athletics.

The enthusiasm around Wilder's bouts was also crucial in reviving heavyweight boxing's popularity among the general public. The division, which has always been the sport's glamorous tier, had lost some of its appeal in the years before Wilder's rise. His electrifying performances and ability to knock out opponents pulled fans who might have been drawn to other combat sports towards heavyweight boxing.

The way that Wilder tackled the business aspect of boxing is indicative of his influence. He intentionally pursued well-known opponents, displaying a readiness to take on formidable opponents. This way of thinking not only kept fans amused but also increased the heavyweight division's general level of competition. By seeking out the greatest bouts available, Wilder demonstrated his dedication to the real spirit of the sport and strengthened his reputation as a real fighter.

The discussions and issues surrounding his defeat by Tyson Fury served to further solidify his legacy narrative. Their contests generated discussions beyond the boxing world, encompassing topics ranging from scoring nuances to fight dynamics. His capacity to pique spectators' curiosity and hold them in debate about the sport cemented his influence on the boxing scene.

Wilder will leave behind a complex legacy as he pursues his career. For present and future generations of boxers, his accomplishments, failures, and the way he behaved himself during his career will be an inspiration and cause for thought. Within the ever-changing realm of professional sports, Deontay Wilder's legacy extends beyond the belts he took home; it also encompasses his lasting influence on boxing as a whole.

11.1 INFLUENCE ON HEAVYWEIGHT BOXING

Throughout his career, Deontay Wilder made a huge impact on the heavyweight boxing community, which continues to this day. Well-known for his remarkable strength and ability to finish fights by knockout, Wilder added excitement and unpredictability to the heavyweight class.

With one of the greatest knockout ratios in heavyweight boxing history, Wilder has demonstrated his ability to terminate fights with a single, devastating blow. In addition to providing fans with entertainment, this fighting style has given the heavyweight division a distinctive new facet. His highlight-reel knockouts attracted a lot of attention and helped the heavyweight class gain popularity again.

The story of American heavyweight boxing was also influenced by the rising stardom of the natives of Alabama. Foreign fighters ruled the heavyweight scene for years, but Wilder's victory gave American heavyweights a boost in popularity. His magnetic charm and exuberant demeanour beyond the arena further won him over supporters and contributed to the development of his brand.

A key component of Wilder's influence on heavyweight boxing is his trilogy with Tyson Fury. The rivalry enthralled fans around the world due to the drama and suspense in each bout. Their contentious draw in their first meeting laid the groundwork for other bouts that brought in massive pay-per-view crowds and raised the heavyweight division's profile internationally.

But it's important to recognize the criticism and difficulties that Wilder encountered throughout his career, especially following his first defeat by Fury in a professional match. The ensuing court cases and public arguments complicated his legacy further. Nevertheless, Wilder's impact endures despite all obstacles.

Wilder's unconventional style, typified by his potent

right hand, has propelled heavyweights forward in terms of technical prowess. His accomplishments have shown that, even in a time when boxing has changed to favour technical skill, a powerful knockout artist can captivate audiences and elevate a fighter's career.

As Wilder's career develops, he will continue to shape the heavyweight class. Whether he makes a comeback to the top of the sport or not, his influence on the boxing scene is already well-established, and his strong punches will live on in the memory of boxing fans for years to come.

The influence that Wilder has had on heavyweight boxing goes beyond his fights. His journey from playing basketball to boxing, where he started late, demonstrates the potential of sheer power and athleticism in the heavyweight class. This story encourages aspiring fighters to follow their goals, highlighting that success in the sport can be achieved through unusual routes.

Known by many as the "Bronze Bomber," Wilder raised awareness of the value of having a strong heavyweight presence in boxing in addition to his own career. His fights with other elite contenders and winners reignited interest in the division and created a favourable atmosphere for a number of thrilling matchups. Wilder's record-breaking run of title defences is clear evidence of his devotion to his art and his desire to win a world championship. His accomplishments, which included winning the WBC heavyweight title, made him a formidable opponent and a symbol of the future of American heavyweight boxing.

Wilder's ability to finish contests has impacted the marketing and promotion of heavyweight bouts. One of the main selling points for Wilder's fights was the expectation of seeing a knockout, which added to the spectacle of big-name boxing matches. Promoters have altered how heavyweight fights are showcased, focusing on the knockout potential to emphasise the explosive characteristics of the heavyweight category.

Wilder further cements his legacy by willingly taking on difficult tasks, such as competing against formidable opponents like Tyson Fury and Luis Ortiz. His unwavering courage in facing the best in the division proved his dedication to leaving a lasting legacy and raised the bar for heavyweight boxing's general level of competition.

Even though Wilder has experienced setbacks in his later career, his tenacity and will to rise to the top highlight how unpredictable the boxing world can be. Whether he makes a comeback or not, Deontay Wilder's impact on heavyweight boxing will go down in history as a time of power, excitement, and resuscitation of interest in a division that holds great historical significance for the sport of boxing.

11.2 CONTRIBUTION TO THE SPORT

Throughout his career, boxing's former heavyweight champion, Deontay Wilder, has made a great deal of contribution to the sport. Renowned for his remarkable strength and ability to finish fights, Wilder introduced a distinctive approach to the heavyweight class that drew admirers from all around the world.

Wilder's remarkable knockout record is among his greatest accomplishments. He has had one of the greatest knockout ratios in heavyweight history for the majority of his career. Known as the "Bronze Bomber," his devastating right hand became his signature weapon, resulting in exciting and dramatic endings in many of his battles.

The heavyweight class saw a surge in enthusiasm and interest in boxing with the ascent of Wilder. His rise through the ranks and victory in the 2015 WBC title gave the division, previously dominated by a small number of well-known names, a dynamic new face. His arrival ushered in an age of uncertainty and excitement, as fans eagerly awaited the spectacle of his spectacular fights.

Wilder's influence went beyond his on-ring exploits; he also helped to revive and promote the heavyweight class. His flamboyant demeanour, candid outlook, and readiness to compete in high-profile bouts helped heavyweight boxing experience a renaissance. While Wilder was the champion, the heavyweight class experienced a rise in popularity, as it is sometimes regarded as the highest level of the sport.

In the sport, Wilder was also instrumental in dismantling barriers and dispelling myths. As the heavyweight champion of African American descent, he inspired a new generation of boxers by serving as an inspirational role model for ambitious athletes. His tenacity and success in the ring served as an example of the value of tenacity and diligence.

But it's important to recognize the controversy that surrounded Wilder's career—especially in light of his well-publicised fights against Tyson Fury. The back-and-forth rivalry between them and the surprising turns their matches took added mystery to Wilder's legacy and highlighted the drama and unpredictable nature of the game.

The boxing world has greatly benefited from Deontay Wilder's numerous contributions. Deontay Wilder's impact on the promotion and popularity of the heavyweight class, in addition to his remarkable knockout power and exciting contests, forever marks the history of boxing. His path, successes, and setbacks have made a lasting impression on the sport and guaranteed him a spot among the greatest heavyweights of his time. Wilder's commitment to giving back to the community was a reflection of his love for the sport. He participated in a number of charity endeavours outside of the ring, such as youth programs and projects that empower marginalised populations. This facet of his persona revealed a more comprehensive comprehension of his public persona and the constructive impact he might provide outside of the boxing world.

Wilder demonstrated his character by bouncing back from setbacks. In 2020, after suffering his first professional defeat at the hands of Tyson Fury, he showed admirable character by showing a will to overcome the setback and taking the loss in stride. This fighter's tenacity moved fans, demonstrating the mental toughness required to weather the highs and lows of a professional boxing career.

Wilder's rise to prominence in the world boxing arena showcases his global influence. Due to the attention his battles have garnered from fans worldwide, the sport has become more globalised. His readiness to fight foreign opponents in high-profile matches cemented his reputation as a global boxing evangelist.

Along with his achievements in the ring, one of the most important contributions to the growth of the sport was Wilder's public appearances and media engagements. He took on the persona of a showman, using style and fascinating storytelling to advertise his fights. This skill at marketing gave his fights an entertaining element that attracted casual spectators and improved the entire spectacle of his shows.

Deontay Wilder had an indisputable overall contribution to boxing, despite difficulties and controversy in the latter half of his career. His effect is evident in the records he broke, the titles he won, and the overall impact he had on the boxing scene. Regardless of whether he pursues a rematch or looks into new chances, Wilder's legacy in the sport will always be an important part of its illustrious past.

CONCLUSION

Through the victories and setbacks of a heavyweight champion, "Deontay Wilder: The Unyielding Warrior" offers an engrossing journey. From his ascent to the top of the boxing world to the difficulties he encountered in the ring, Wilder's unwavering resolve and steadfast spirit are visible throughout his career.

By examining Wilder's devastating knockout power and unconventional methodology, the book explores the subtleties of his unusual fighting technique. By examining the physical and mental toughness needed to succeed in the competitive world of professional boxing, it illuminates the selflessness and commitment that characterise a real fighter.

Beyond the glamour of triumphs, the story also discusses the obstacles that Wilder had to overcome. The champion's fortitude shines through incontrovertible choices and defeats in the ring, serving as a source of motivation for those going through similar struggles. Readers learn more about Wilder's personality and the guy behind the gloves as the chapters turn. The book encapsulates his path and highlights the significance of self-belief, dedication, and tenacity in pursuing greatness.

This examination of Deontay Wilder's life and career not only honours his accomplishments but also humanises the champion, putting him in the shoes of both sports fans and up-and-coming athletes. The narrative goes beyond sporting limits to become a tale of perseverance and the unwavering spirit that characterises a great warrior.

In the end, "Deontay Wilder: The Unyielding Warrior" illustrates the highs and lows of an incredible career and serves as a monument to the lasting legacy of a heavyweight champion. It leaves readers with a deep respect for boxing as a sport and the remarkable people who represent its spirit, making a lasting impression on the history of the sweet discipline.